FIBROID DIET

Fibroid meal plan preparation

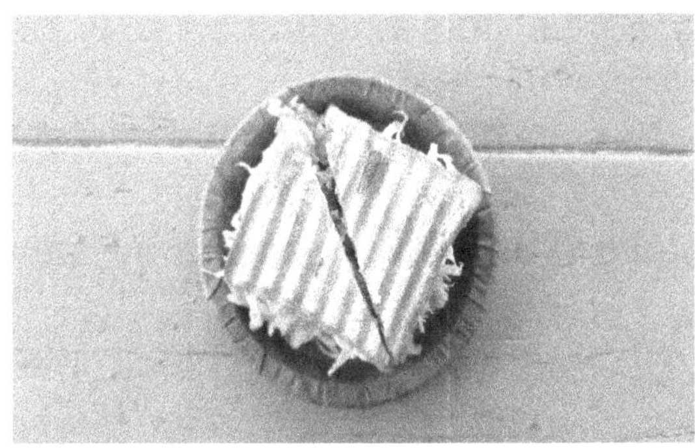

MAURICE VINCENT

TABLE OF CONTENT

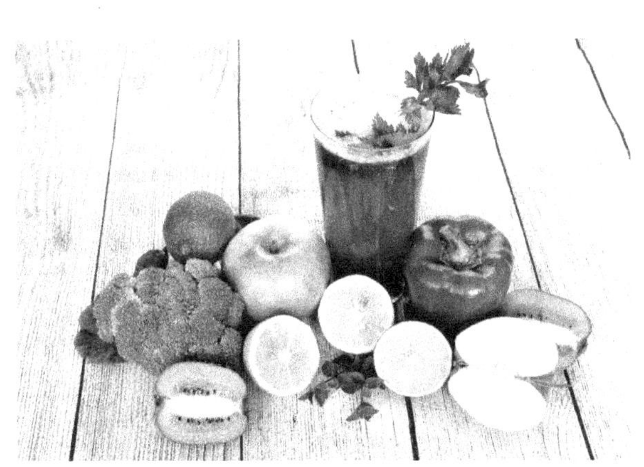

INTRODUCTION

My name is Maurice Vincent.

A meal plan for individuals with fibroids should focus on a balanced and nutrient-rich diet that may help manage symptoms. It's important to note that dietary changes alone may not cure or eliminate fibroids, but they can potentially contribute to overall well-being.

I went into this because I felt I could help people with food ideas. I realize people repeat the same foods every day and over time, the foods get boring. I thought of the idea of drafting food plans for people, giving them different foods to try out all day in a week. A well-balanced healthy food plan.

After drafting the food plans for families, I extended them to weight loss. I understand the struggle that comes with losing weight and how most of the foods online are difficult to come by. So,

I devised a means to get cheaper and available foods for people. Knowing that most people would also love to add weight, I ventured into that as well. I was a skinny female and I got bullied and body-shamed a lot while growing up, but in a year, I made a difference in the foods I ate, hehehehe, I am no longer skinny.

If you would like to add weight, lose weight, or have healthy food ideas for you and your family, or for your kids who are picky eaters, I suggest you give me a try.

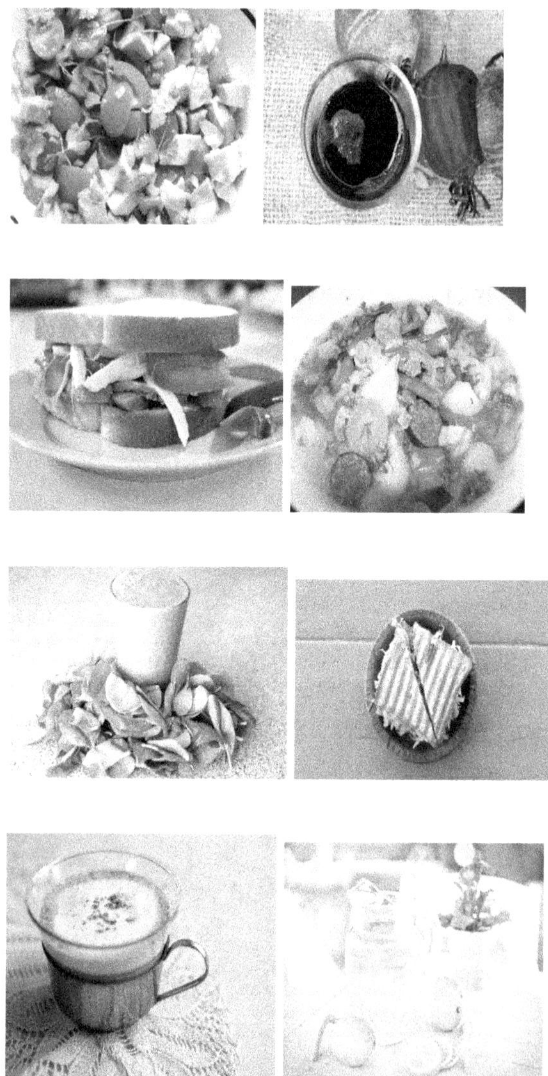

CHAPTER 1

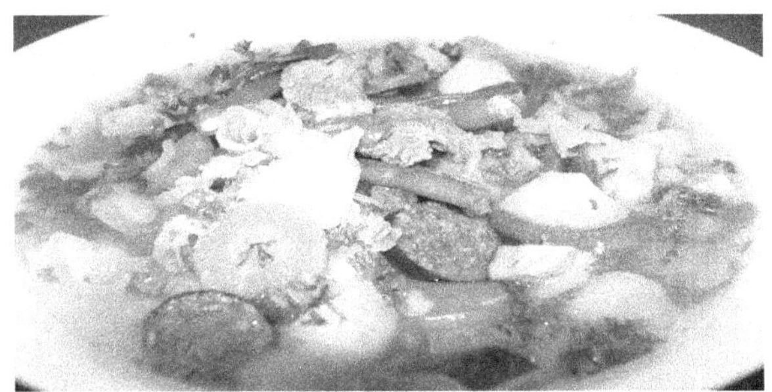

<u>BASIC DEFINITION OF FIBROID</u>

Fibroids, medically known as uterine leiomyomas or myomas, are noncancerous growths that develop in the uterus. These tumours are made of muscle cells and fibrous tissue and can vary in size, ranging from small and undetectable to large enough to cause significant discomfort.

<u>THE CAUSES OF FIBROID</u>

The precise cause of fibroids remains unclear, but various factors may contribute to their development. Hormonal fluctuations, particularly elevated estrogen levels, genetic predisposition, and family history are believed to play a role in their formation. Additionally, other factors like age, ethnicity, and obesity may influence their occurrence.

<u>**SYMPTOMS**</u>

Fibroids can manifest with a range of symptoms, and their severity varies among individuals. Common symptoms include:

<u>Menstrual Changes:</u> Heavier or prolonged menstrual periods, irregular periods, and pelvic pain.

Pelvic Discomfort: Pressure or pain in the lower abdomen or pelvic region.

Frequent Urination: Enlarged fibroids may press against the

bladder, causing increased frequency of urination.

Backache or Leg Pains: Large fibroids can exert pressure on surrounding organs and nerves, leading to back or leg discomfort. Pain during Intercourse: Fibroids may cause pain or discomfort during sexual intercourse.

PREVENTION

While it may not be possible to prevent fibroids entirely, certain lifestyle choices and interventions may help manage their impact:

Healthy Diet: Maintain a well-balanced diet rich in fruits, vegetables, and whole grains.

Regular Exercise: Engage in regular physical activity to manage weight and promote overall well-being.

Limit Alcohol and Caffeine: Moderate alcohol consumption and reduce caffeine intake.

Regular Check-ups: Attend routine gynaecological check-ups for early detection and management.

AGE RANGE

Fibroids are most commonly diagnosed during a woman's reproductive years, typically between the ages of 30 and 40. However, they can occur at any age, and some women may not experience noticeable symptoms. As women approach menopause, hormonal changes oftcn lead to a natural reduction in the size and impact of fibroids. It's crucial for individuals experiencing symptoms to consult with a healthcare professional for proper diagnosis and guidance on appropriate management strategies.

CHAPTER 2

FIBROID MEAL PLAN PREPARATION

A fibroid meal plan focuses on dietary choices that may help manage symptoms associated with uterine fibroids. While there's no one-size-fits-all solution, adopting a nutrient-rich and well-balanced diet can contribute to overall well-being and potentially alleviate some discomfort associated with fibroids. It's important to note that dietary changes should be discussed with a healthcare professional, and the meal plan is just one aspect of a holistic approach to managing fibroids. In this book, I have been able to provide diverse meal plans and easy ways to prepare the meals.

KEY PRINCIPALS OF A FIBROID MEAL PLAN

Nutrient-Rich Foods: Emphasize whole foods, such as fruits, vegetables, lean proteins, and whole grains, to ensure a diverse range of essential nutrients.

Fiber Intake: Include high-fiber foods like whole grains, legumes, and vegetables to support digestive health and hormonal balance.

Healthy Fats: Incorporate sources of healthy fats, such as avocados, nuts, seeds, and olive oil, which can have anti-inflammatory properties.

Iron-rich foods: Address potential anaemia related to heavy menstrual bleeding by including iron-rich foods like lean meats, spinach, and legumes.

Hydration: Stay well-hydrated with water and herbal teas to support overall health and hydration.

Limit Processed Foods: Minimize intake of processed foods, added sugars, and unhealthy fats to promote general well-being.

Remember, while a fibroid meal plan may contribute to symptom management, it's part of a comprehensive approach that may also include medical interventions, lifestyle modifications, and professional guidance. Always seek professional advice before making significant changes to your diet or healthcare regimen.

FIBROID MEAL PLAN

Designing a fibroid meal plan involves emphasizing nutrient-rich foods that may support overall health and potentially alleviate symptoms. A balanced approach includes incorporating fruits, vegetables, whole grains, lean proteins, and healthy fats. Key considerations for a fibroid-friendly meal plan include: This Meal plan consists of a variety of meals and drinks that can help manage Fibroid:-

Turmeric Tea

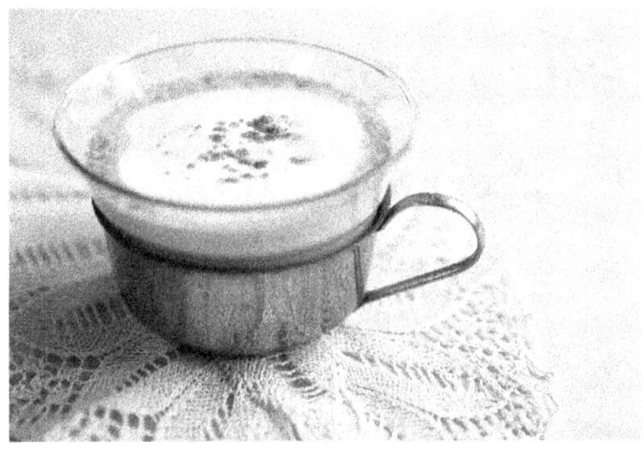

Turmeric tea, derived from the turmeric root, is often lauded for its potential health benefits due to its active compound curcumin. While research on turmeric's specific effects on fibroids is limited, some potential benefits may be associated with its anti-inflammatory and antioxidant properties. Here are the benefits of Tumeric tea*:-*

Anti-Inflammatory Effects:

Curcumin, the active ingredient in turmeric, is known for its anti-inflammatory properties. Inflammation is believed to play a role in various health conditions, including fibroids. Consuming turmeric tea may help reduce inflammation in the body.

Antioxidant Properties:

Turmeric is rich in antioxidants, which can help combat oxidative stress. Antioxidants play a role in supporting overall health and may contribute to reducing cellular damage.

Hormonal Balance:

Some studies suggest that curcumin may influence hormonal balance by modulating estrogen levels. Since fibroids are hormone-sensitive growths, this property might have potential benefits in managing symptoms.

Pain Relief:

Turmeric's anti-inflammatory effects may contribute to pain relief. Women with fibroids may experience pelvic pain, and turmeric tea might help alleviate some discomfort.

Menstrual Regulation:

Some studies propose that curcumin may have regulatory effects on the menstrual cycle. For women with fibroids, this could potentially contribute to managing menstrual irregularities.

Overall Well-Being:

Turmeric tea is a low-calorie beverage that can be part of a healthy diet. Staying hydrated with herbal teas like turmeric tea can contribute to overall well-being.

It's crucial to note that while turmeric tea might offer potential benefits, it is not a substitute for professional medical advice and treatment. Fibroids vary in size and symptoms, and individual responses to dietary changes can differ. A comprehensive approach to managing fibroids may involve a combination of medical interventions, lifestyle modifications, and individualized care.

Ingredients for Tumeric Tea :

1 cup of almond milk

2 spoons of turmeric powder

1 spoon of ginger powder or grated ginger

1 spoon of black pepper

1 spoon of honey

1 spoon of cinnamon

1 cup of tiger nuts (alternative)

PREPARATIONS:

Soak the tiger nuts overnight and blend the next morning or soak in hot water for 10mins before blending.

DIRECTIONS:

1. Blend the tiger nuts until very smooth using warm water

2. Sieve, throw away the shaft and keep the milk aside.

3. Add a spoonful of turmeric powder and ginger powder to the warm tiger nuts milk.

4. Stir and drink.

These directions are for tiger nuts, however, if you are not using tiger nuts,

1. Just combine the almond milk, turmeric powder, powdered ginger, black pepper, honey and

cinnamon in a blender and blend till very smooth.

<u>**TIP:**</u>

1. Black pepper is very important to use in this drink as it makes your body absorb the turmeric faster.

Ginger Tea

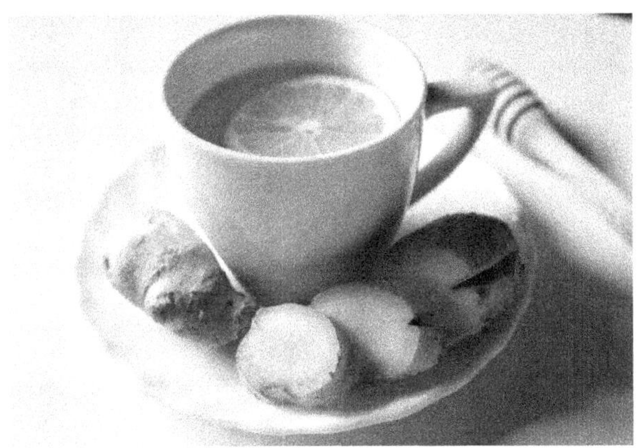

Ginger tea is appreciated for its potential health benefits, but specific evidence regarding its direct effects on fibroids is limited. However, ginger does possess certain properties that might contribute to overall well-being, and some potential benefits could be relevant to fibroid management:

Anti-Inflammatory Properties:

Ginger contains compounds with anti-inflammatory effects. Chronic inflammation is associated with various health conditions, and reducing inflammation might have a positive impact on symptoms related to fibroids.

Pain Relief:

Ginger is traditionally known for its analgesic (pain-relieving) properties. Women with fibroids may experience pelvic pain, and ginger tea might offer some relief.

Digestive Health:

Ginger tea can promote digestive health by easing nausea and potentially reducing bloating. This may be beneficial for individuals experiencing digestive discomfort related to fibroids.

Blood Circulation:

Ginger is believed to improve blood circulation. This may have potential benefits for women with fibroids, as improved circulation is associated with overall health.

Antioxidant Content:

Ginger is rich in antioxidants, which can help combat

oxidative stress. Antioxidants play a role in supporting overall health and may contribute to reducing cellular damage.

Hormonal Balance:

Some studies suggest that ginger may influence hormonal balance, including modulating estrogen levels. Since fibroids are hormone-sensitive, this property might have potential benefits.

Menstrual Symptom Relief:

Ginger tea might help alleviate symptoms associated with menstruation, such as menstrual cramps. Women with fibroids may find relief from certain menstrual symptoms.

Warmth and Comfort:

Warm beverages like ginger tea can provide comfort, especially during times of menstrual discomfort. The soothing effect may contribute to a sense of well-being.

It's essential to approach ginger tea or any herbal remedies as complementary to professional medical advice. Fibroids can vary in size and symptoms, and individual responses to herbal treatments can differ. A holistic approach to fibroid management often involves a combination of medical interventions, lifestyle adjustments, and personalized care.

Ingredients for Ginger Tea:

2 ginger root (peeled and grated)

1 spoon of honey

1 lemon or lime (optional)

DIRECTIONS:

1. Boil 1 cup of water

2. Add the grated ginger in a cup.

3. Add 1 spoon of honey to the cup.

4. Add a slice of lemon or lime OR squeeze the lemon juice or lime into the cup.

5. Pour the boiling water into the cup.

6. Leave for 5mins

7. Serve.

Lemon Drink:

This cleanses or detoxifies your system. Take every morning on an empty stomach.

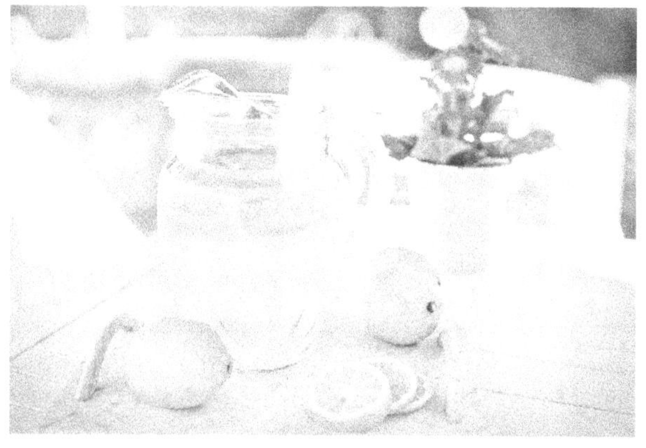

Lemon tea itself may not have direct evidence supporting its effects on fibroids, it can be a refreshing and healthful beverage that provides some potential benefits. It's important to note that fibroids vary in size and symptoms, and individual responses to dietary changes can differ. Here are some general benefits associated with lemon tea that might contribute to overall well-being:

Vitamin C Boost:

Lemons are rich in vitamin C, a powerful antioxidant that supports the immune system and may contribute to overall health.

Hydration:

Staying well-hydrated is crucial for overall health, and lemon tea can be a flavorful and hydrating alternative to sugary beverages.

Digestive Aid:

Lemon tea, especially when consumed warm, may act as a gentle digestive aid and help alleviate bloating or indigestion.

Alkalizing Properties:

While lemons are acidic, they have alkalizing effects on the body. Some proponents of alkaline diets suggest that maintaining a slightly alkaline environment may be beneficial for health.

Flavor without Calories:

Lemon tea can add flavour to your drink without adding significant calories, making it a healthy beverage choice.

<u>***Refreshing and Comforting:***</u>

The aroma and taste of lemon can be refreshing and comforting, providing a pleasant sensory experience.

While lemon tea is generally safe for most people, it's important to remember that individual responses to dietary changes vary. Lemon tea can be part of a balanced and varied diet, but it should not be considered a standalone treatment for fibroids.

Ingredient for Lemon Tea:

1 Lemon

3 spoons of Apple Cider Vinegar

DIRECTION:

Squeeze the juice of 1 lemon into 1 cup

of warm water.

Sandwich/ Toast Bread

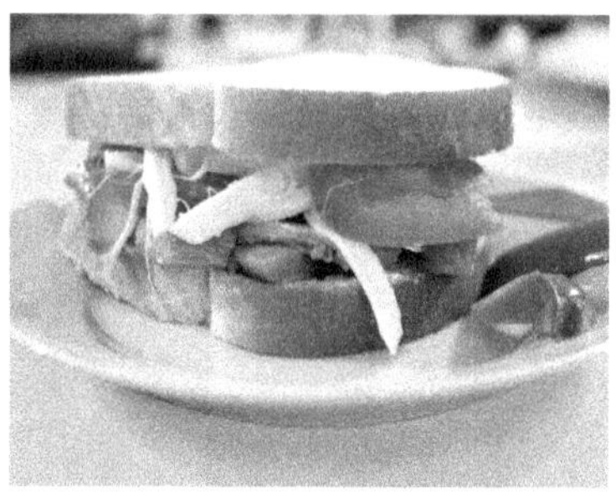

<u>*Ingredients*</u>*:*

4 slices of Wheat bread

1 tomato

Lettuce

2 boiled eggs

1 boiled fish

PREPARATION

1. Toast the bread, but if you don't have a sandwich maker, you can skip this step.

2. Apply 1 spoon of butter on the bread.

3. Place your already-washed lettuce on top of the bread.

4. Then your thinly sliced tomatoes.

5. Followed by the sliced eggs.

6. Onions.

7. And the boiled fish, if you will be using it.

8. Cover with another bread.

9. Serve.

Guacamole

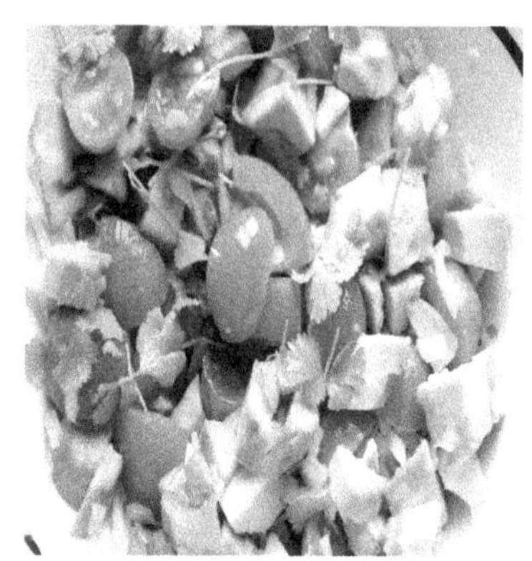

Ingredients:

3 avocado

1 tomato

1 onion

Salt

Coriander leaf (curry leaf)

PREPARATIONS:

Slice your onions, tomato and leaves.
Set aside.

DIRECTIONS:

1. Mash the avocado in a bowl

2. Pour the sliced onions, tomato and
leaf inside and stir

3. Add salt for taste.

4. Eat with Boiled Potatoes and plantain.

Spinach Smoothie

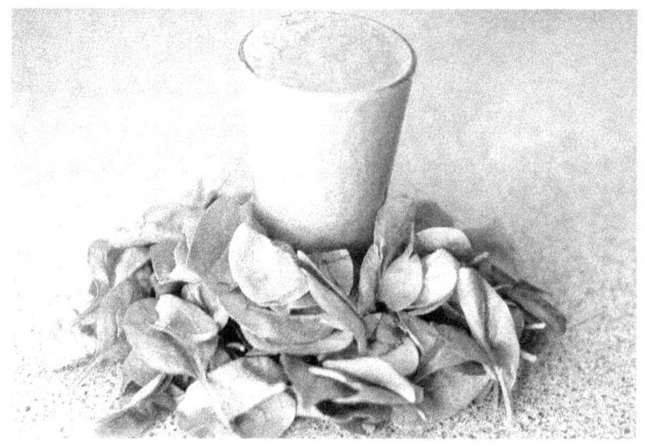

Spinach is a nutrient-dense leafy green vegetable that provides various health benefits. Including spinach in your diet as part of an overall nutritious and balanced approach may contribute to your well-being. Here are some potential benefits associated with spinach and its nutrients:

Iron-Rich Source:

Spinach is a good source of iron, which is important for individuals with fibroids who may experience heavy menstrual bleeding and be at risk of anaemia.

Fibre Content:

Spinach is high in fibre, which supports digestive health. Adequate fibre intake is beneficial for overall well-being.

Vitamins and Minerals:

Spinach is rich in vitamins A, C, and K, as well as minerals like potassium and magnesium. These nutrients play essential roles in various bodily functions.

Antioxidant Properties:

Spinach contains antioxidants, including beta-carotene, lutein, and zeaxanthin. Antioxidants help combat oxidative stress and may contribute to overall health.

Anti-Inflammatory Potential:

Certain compounds in spinach, such as flavonoids and carotenoids, may have anti-inflammatory effects. Chronic inflammation is associated with various health conditions.

Regulation of Hormones:

Some studies suggest that a diet rich in fruits and vegetables, including spinach, may have a positive impact on hormonal balance. Since fibroids are hormone-sensitive, this balance may be beneficial.

It's important to emphasize that a nutritious diet is essential for overall health.

Ingredients:

2 handful of spinach

1 banana

1 lime (extract the juice)

<u>*DIRECTIONS:*</u>

1. Combine all ingredients and blend till smooth.

2. Add ½ glass of water.

3. Blend again for 3mins.

4. Serve.

Watermelon Smoothie

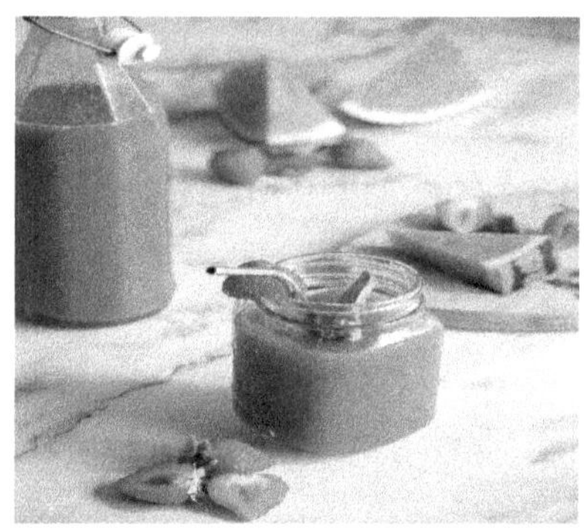

<u>Benefits of Watermelon Smooth</u>

<u>*Hydration:*</u>

Watermelon has a high water content, contributing to hydration. Staying well-hydrated is essential for overall health.

Vitamins and Antioxidants:

Watermelon is a good source of vitamins A and C, as well as antioxidants like lycopene. These nutrients support immune function and combat oxidative stress.

Low in Calories:

Watermelon is relatively low in calories, making it a refreshing and guilt-free snack option.

Natural Sweetness:

Watermelon's natural sweetness can satisfy cravings for sweets without added sugars, contributing to a balanced diet.

Digestive Health:

The fibre content in watermelon, although not extremely high, can contribute to digestive health.

Ingredients:

Cold watermelon

1 orange

PREPARATIONS:

Open the watermelon and deseed it. Cut

into sizeable chunks

Take out the seeds from the orange.

<u>DIRECTION:</u>

Add the watermelon in a blender.

Squeeze out the orange juice, and add

½ or ¾ cup of water. Do not make it too

thick

Banana Smoothie

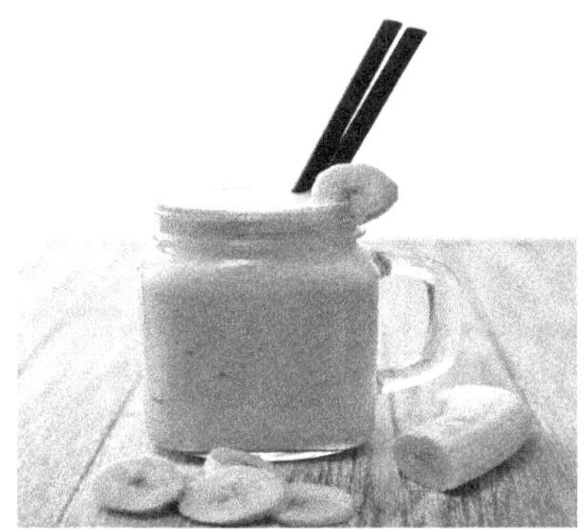

<u>Benefits of Banana smooth</u>

Bananas are a good source of essential nutrients, including potassium, vitamin C, vitamin B6, and dietary fibre. These nutrients play crucial roles in various bodily functions.

Energy Boost:

Bananas are a convenient and portable snack that provides a quick energy boost due to their carbohydrate content.

Anti-Inflammatory Properties:

Bananas contain certain compounds with potential anti-inflammatory effects. Chronic inflammation is associated with various health conditions.

<u>Blood Sugar Regulation:</u>

The natural sugars in bananas, combined with fibre, may contribute to stable blood sugar levels, making them a suitable snack option for those managing blood sugar.

While bananas can be part of a healthy diet, it's crucial to approach dietary choices for managing fibroids as part of a comprehensive strategy.

Ingredients:

3 bananas

Unsweetened yoghurt

Milk (Liquid Preferably but you can use powdered milk)

DIRECTIONS:

1. Combine all ingredients in a blender.

2. Blend till smooth.

3. If you are using powdered milk, add water to have a creamy smoothie.

4. Blend for 3 -5mins.

5. Add more water milk or yoghurt if it is

too thick.

6. Serve

Broccoli Smoothie

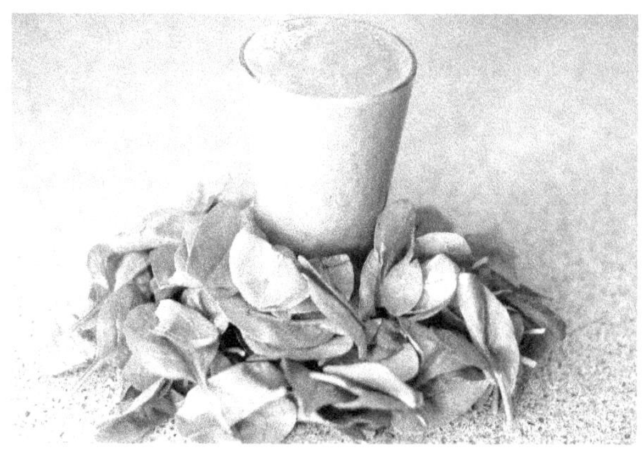

<u>Benefits of Broccoli smooth</u>

<u>*Nutrient Density:*</u>

Broccoli is rich in essential nutrients, including vitamin C, vitamin K, folate, and dietary fibre. These nutrients play crucial roles in maintaining overall health.

Antioxidant Properties:

Broccoli contains antioxidants, such as sulforaphane and quercetin, which help combat oxidative stress and inflammation. Chronic inflammation is associated with various health conditions.

Detoxification Support:

Compounds in broccoli, particularly glucosinolates, are known to support the body's natural detoxification processes.

Fibre Content:

The fibre in broccoli contributes to digestive health by promoting regular bowel movements and supporting a healthy gut microbiome.

<u>***Potential Hormonal Balance:***</u>

Some studies suggest that cruciferous vegetables, including broccoli, may influence estrogen metabolism. Since fibroids are hormone-sensitive, this property may have potential benefits

<u>***Ingredients***</u>

1 banana

1 cup of low-fat milk or 1 cup of Greek or Unsweetened Yoghurt

A handful of broccoli

DIRECTIONS:

1. In a blender, combine all ingredients.

Add ½ cup of water.

2. Blend till smooth.

3. Serve.

Kale Smoothie

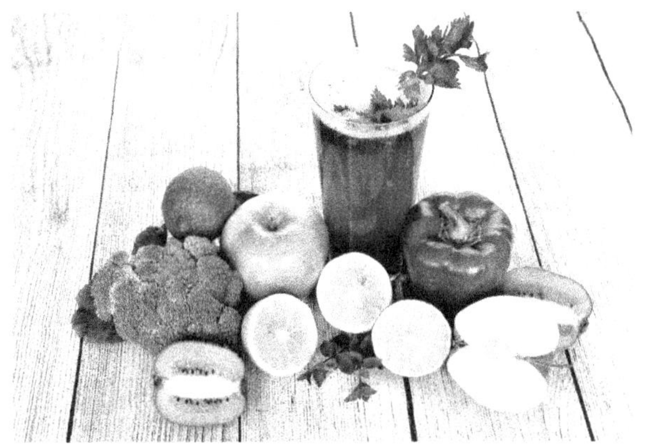

Kale is rich in essential nutrients, including vitamins A, C, and K, and minerals such as calcium and iron.

Antioxidant Content:

Kale contains antioxidants, such as flavonoids and carotenoids, which help combat oxidative stress and support cellular health.

Anti-Inflammatory Properties:

Compounds in kale, including glucosinolates and quercetin, may have anti-inflammatory effects, potentially benefiting overall health.

<u>Fibre Content</u>:

Kale is high in fibre, promoting digestive health by supporting regular bowel movements and aiding in digestion.

<u>Detoxification Support</u>:

Kale contains sulfur-containing compounds that may support the body's natural detoxification processes.

Ingredient:

1 cup of pineapple (small pineapple)

1 cup of coconut water

1 cold banana

2 handfuls of kale (spinach)

PREPARATIONS:

1. Combine all ingredients: chopped pineapple, coconut water, banana and kale, in a blender.

2. Blend for 5mins.

3. Drink

Beetroot Juice Booster

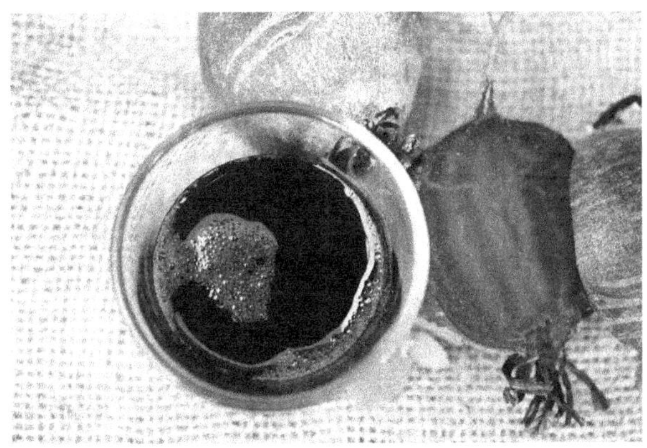

Antioxidant Content:

Beetroot is rich in antioxidants, including betalains and polyphenols, which help combat oxidative stress and inflammation.

Anti-Inflammatory Properties:

Compounds in beetroot, such as betalains, may have anti-inflammatory effects, potentially benefiting overall health.

Detoxification Support:

The betalains in beetroot have been studied for their potential support in the body's natural detoxification processes.

<u>**Potential Hormonal Balance:**</u>

Some studies suggest that the antioxidants in beetroot may have a positive impact on hormonal balance. Since fibroids are hormone-sensitive, this property may have potential benefits

<u>*Ingredients:*</u>

2 ginger heads

3 beetroots

1 lemon

1 apple

4 ice cubes

PREPARATIONS:

Cut the beetroot into sizeable sizes.

Dice the apple into small sizes

Squeeze out the juice from the lemon

Grate the ginger

DIRECTIONS:

1. Combine all ingredients in a blender.

2. Blend till very smooth.

3. Serve.

Avocado Shakes

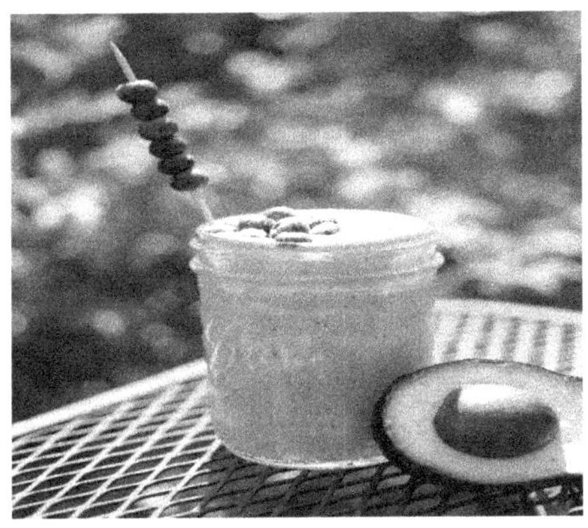

<u>Nutrient Density:</u>

Avocados are a good source

of   essential   nutrients,

including vitamins E, C, B6,

folate,   potassium,   and

dietary fibre.

Antioxidant Content:

Avocados contain antioxidants, including lutein and zeaxanthin, which help combat oxidative stress and support cellular health.

Anti-Inflammatory Properties:

Some compounds in avocados, such as carotenoids and polyphenols, have potential anti-inflammatory effects, which may be beneficial for overall health.

Blood Sugar Regulation:

The monounsaturated fats and fibre in avocados may contribute to stable blood sugar levels, making them a suitable option for those managing blood sugar.

Digestive Health:

Avocados contain soluble and insoluble fibre, promoting digestive health by supporting regular bowel movements.

Hormonal Balance:

While more research is needed, some studies suggest that a diet rich in certain nutrients found in avocados may positively influence hormonal balance.

While avocados can be part of a nutritious diet, it's crucial to approach dietary choices for managing fibroids as part of a comprehensive strategy, dietary adjustments, and lifestyle modifications. Remember that individual responses to specific foods can vary, and avocados should be consumed as part of a balanced and varied diet.

Ingredients:

1 or 2 cold avocados

1 cold banana

1 spoon of honey

½ cup of water or milk or yoghurt

DIRECTIONS:

Combine all ingredients: avocado, banana, honey, and your choice of liquid in a blender.

Cabbage Soup

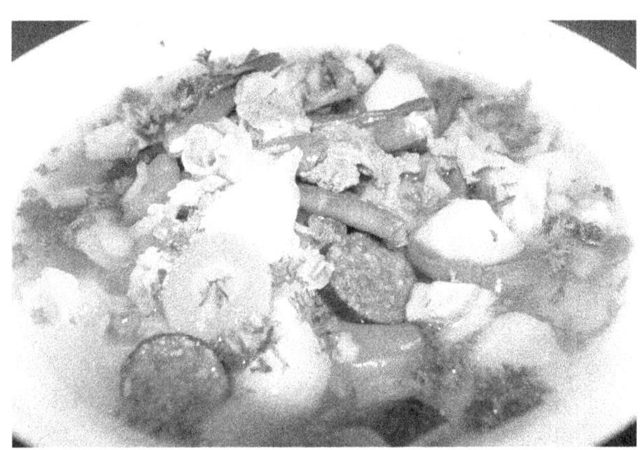

<u>BENEFITS OF CABBAGE</u>

<u>Antioxidant Properties</u>:

Cabbage contains antioxidants, including flavonoids and polyphenols, which help combat oxidative stress and support cellular health.

Anti-Inflammatory Effects:

Compounds in cabbage, such as glucosinolates and anthocyanins, may have anti-inflammatory effects, potentially benefiting overall health.

Detoxification Support:

Cabbage contains sulfur-containing compounds that may support the body's natural detoxification processes.

Potential Hormonal Balance:

Cruciferous vegetables like cabbage contain indole-3-carbinol, which has been studied for its potential influence on estrogen metabolism. Since fibroids are hormone-sensitive, this property may have potential benefits.

<u>*Ingredients:*</u>

1 onion

1 head of cabbage

2 carrots

2 cloves of garlic

2 bay leaves

1kg of turkey

2 tablespoons of tomato paste

Handful of spinach

<u>*PREPARATIONS:*</u>

Slice Onions and set aside.

Grate your garlic and set aside.

Dice the carrots. Chop the cabbage and

celery stalks

Season turkey with onions, salt, pepper

and stock cubes. Set broth aside

DIRECTIONS:

1. Combine all vegetables in a pot.

2. Add the tomato paste, broth from the seasoned turkey, bay leaves, seasoning, and pepper and stir to combine.

3. Cover and cook for 20mins.

4. Once cooked, add spinach and cook for 5mins more.

5. Turn off burner.

Serve.

Garlic Tea

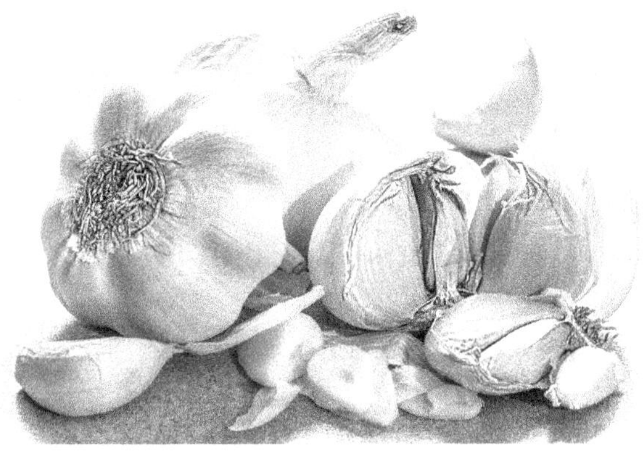

Garlic has been studied for its potential health benefits, but there is limited specific evidence on its direct effects on fibroids. Garlic contains bioactive compounds, including allicin, which is known for its antimicrobial and anti-inflammatory properties. Here are some potential benefits associated with garlic that might contribute to overall well-being:

Anti-Inflammatory Properties:

Garlic has been recognized for its anti-inflammatory effects, which may help reduce inflammation in the body. Chronic inflammation is associated with various health conditions.

Antioxidant Content:

Garlic contains antioxidants that can help combat oxidative stress.

Antioxidants play a role in supporting overall health.

Potential Hormonal Balance:

Some studies suggest that garlic may have a modulating effect on hormones, including estrogen. Since fibroids are hormone-sensitive, this property may have potential benefits.

Immune System Support:

Garlic is known for its immune-boosting properties, and regular consumption may contribute to overall immune system health.

Cardiovascular Health:

Garlic has been studied for its potential benefits in supporting heart health, including the ability to help regulate blood pressure and cholesterol levels.

Anti-Microbial Properties:

Garlic possesses antimicrobial properties that may help fight against certain infections.

It's important to note that while garlic tea might offer potential health benefits, Individual responses to specific foods or remedies can vary, and garlic tea should be consumed as part of a balanced and varied diet.

Ingredients for Garlic Tea:

2 garlic (peeled and grated)

1 spoon of honey

1 lemon or lime (optional)

DIRECTIONS:

1. Boil 1 cup of water

2. Add the grated garlic in a cup.

3. Add 1 spoon of honey to the cup.

4. Add a slice of lemon or lime OR squeeze the lemon juice or lime into the cup.

5. Pour the boiling water into the cup.

6. Leave for 5mins

7. Serve

<u>*CONCLUSION*</u>

Crafting a fibroid meal plan involves thoughtful consideration of nutrient-rich foods that may positively impact overall health and potentially alleviate fibroid symptoms. Focusing on a diverse array of colorful fruits and vegetables, incorporating whole grains, lean proteins, and healthy fats creates a foundation for a balanced and nutritious diet. These dietary choices aim to provide essential vitamins, minerals, antioxidants, and fibre, contributing to digestive health, hormonal balance, and overall well-being.

 Additionally, staying well-hydrated with water and herbal teas is essential for supporting bodily functions. Striving guidance from healthcare professionals, such as a gynaecologist or registered dietitian, ensures a personalized and effective strategy. By embracing a balanced fibroid-friendly meal plan, promoting both physical and emotional well-being.